7 PRESCRIPTION DRUG BIOHACKS

Hot Bio-hacks That Can Help You Increase Your Medication's Effectiveness

Olivia L. Young, PhD, PMHNP-BC, MAT-C

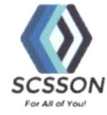

SCSSON
For All of You!

7 Prescription Drug Bio-hacks
Copyright © 2019 by Olivia L. Young - All Rights Reserved.

All rights reserved. No part of this book may be reproduced in any form or by any electronic or mechanical means including information storage and retrieval systems, without permission in writing from the author. The only exception is by a reviewer, who may quote short excerpts in a review.

Cover designed
by
Adam@perfect_designs, Nigeria

NP Dr. Olivia L. Young
Visit my webpage at www.scsson.com/NPDrYoung

Produced in the United States of America

First Published: Dec 2019
Scsson Publishing Company

DISCLAIMERS

7 Prescription Drug Biohacks is intended solely for informational and educational purposes, and is not meant for use as medical advice. If you have questions about your health, please talk with your health care provider.

The opinions expressed herein are the author's own. Some of the opinions expressed may not reflect those held by the publisher.

CONTENTS

Why You Need to Read This Book 1

PART ONE: Introduction and Overview 3

Introduction 4

Biohacking And Taking Prescription Drugs 9

PART TWO: The 7 Biohacks 17

Biohack #1 18

Bio-Hack #2 20

Bio-Hack #3 22

Bio-Hack #4 23

Bio-Hack #5 25

Bio-Hack #6 26

List Of Drug Classes Known To Cause Nutrient Depletion 28

Bio-Hack #7 29

Epilogue 30

PART THREE: Publisher and Author Notes 32

About Scsson 33

About The Author 35

Scsson's Self Care Support Plan 36

May I Ask You A Favor? 37

Free Bio-Hacking Tools On The Internet 38

Send Questions, Send Feedback 39

WHY YOU NEED TO READ THIS BOOK

Do you take prescription medications? If you do, were you told about the side effects and related health problems they can cause? Were you told how to avoid those problems? If your answer to the first question is yes while your answers to the second and third questions are no, you need to read this book.

Even though you take prescription drugs, would you like to improve your health? Did your health care prescriber tell you how you can support and improve your body's biochemistry while taking prescription drugs that damage the body's biochemical processes and metabolic pathways? Were you told how to help strengthen and lengthen your telomeres as part of an antiaging strategy? If your answer to the first question is yes but your answers to the second and third questions are no, you need to read this book.

What You Will Get From Reading This Book

You will get 1) a brief, nontechnical introduction to biohacking, explicit definitions of the terms and ideas that provide the framework for biohacking your prescription drugs, 2) a nontechnical discussion about safe medication administration, 3) a list of 7 great prescription drug biohacks, along with a brief explanation about each, 4) a list of drug classifications whose compounds require biohacking, and 5) links to resources that can help you understand the science involved with each biohack.

Importantly, after reading this book, you will see that you can implement the hacks as part of your own home-based self-help, healthcare regimen. While you may wish to discuss them with your health care provider, the specific health problems caused by prescription drugs are problems that you will likely be able to remediate by biohacking them at home, mostly on your own.

Finally, the biohacks are great evidence-based self care tips about specific activities that you can do to help increase the effectiveness of the prescription drugs. Further, these same activities will also help optimize your health-- and quite probably, your healthy longevity!

PART ONE
INTRODUCTION AND OVERVIEW

INTRODUCTION

Why You May Need to Biohack Your Prescription Drugs

As a wellness oriented advanced practice registered nurse (APRN) who is a board certified psychiatric mental health nurse practitioner (PMHNP-BC), I frequently encounter patients who present with a variety of complaints. Typically, the patients also manifest a variety of dysfunctional lifestyle related disorders (a disorder is a disruption to normal body structure or function) and behaviors. Some of these include eating a lot of fake food, having poor hydration, being chronically exposed to a myriad of toxins, and taking a large number of pharmaceutical and over the counter (OTC) drugs. Many of these individuals are also suffering from side effects that are being caused by the drugs they are taking.

Some of the known drug side effects can present as various kinds of body pains, syndromes, gastrointestinal problems, nervous system problems, and/or other constitutional signs, symptoms, and problems. A syndrome is a collection of signs and symptoms in one area of the body but the specific causal pathology can't be determined. Some of the specific complaints in the above list may be as follows:

Some pain related complaints include having:

- Pain all over
- Pain in the legs

- Back pain
- Joint pain
- Pain when emptying the bladder
- Chest pain

Some of the "other" complaints include having:

- Painful menstruation
- Irregular menstrual cycles
- Burning feeling in sexual organs
- Pain during coitus
- Premature ejaculation
- Erectile dysfunction
- Unintentional weight gain or loss
- High blood pressure or low blood pressure
- Easy bruising

Some gastrointestinal related complaints are about having:

- Stomach pain or spasms
- Nausea
- Vomiting
- Diarrhea
- Constipation
- GI Bloating, excessive gas
- Food intolerance

Some syndrome related complaints are about having:

- TMJ* pain
- Irritable bowel syndrome
- Chronic fatigue syndrome

- Fibromyalgia
- Premenstrual Syndrome (PMS)

*TMJ stands for temporomandibular joint. The TMJ is the place where the upper and lower jaws come together.

Some of the nervous system related complaints are about having:

- Muscle weakness
- Trouble talking
- Dizziness or Fainting
- Double or blurred vision
- Memory problems
- Headaches
- Trouble or pain when walking
- Shakes or tremors

Some nervous system mental health related complaints are about having:

- Anxiety
- Depression
- Anger outbursts
- Sleep problems
- Eating problems
- Loss of appetite problems
- Parkinson like symptoms
- Hyperactivity

So Many Problems and So Little Time

Although patients may faithfully keep the quarterly medication check, follow-up visits typically allowed by their third-party payers, their prescribing or other health care provider will often be clueless as to the cause of the above complaints. The provider is also likely to feel inadequate to address the complaints, and may ignore them or diagnose the patient with the appropriate catch all International Statistical Classification of Diseases and Related Health Problems 10th Revision (ICD-10) code of Somatization Disorder. The term, "disorder" is used in health care to indicate the existence of some type of problem or deviation from the normally expected body structure(s) or function(s).

ICD-10 codes are the alphanumeric codes used by health care providers (HCP), health insurance companies, and public health agencies across the world to indicate the HCP's diagnoses of the type of problem the patient has. Every formally acknowledged disease, disorder, injury, infection, and symptom has its own ICD-10 code. The codes are widely used for everything-- processing health insurance claims, tracking epidemics, and compiling worldwide mortality statistics, to name a few. You can find more about Somatization Disorder code at the online ICD-10 web page. Click here to take a quick look and then bookmark it if you want to be able to study it in more detail later on, by exploring the many links on the page.

Unfortunately, the U.S. health care system operates on an insurance or third-party payer model of paying for health care services. Ultimately, and partially due to the well-known phenomenon of institutional creep, third party payers have become the major determiners of the kind, quantity, and length of health care insureds are allowed. See Break The Health Insurance Habit by Dr. Destiny N Patel ("N" is her middle name) for a more in-depth review of this health and life denying problem.

In its ignorance and/or callous disregard of the sacredness of human life, the current model has created algorithms that presumes individuals with certain characteristics are all essentially the same. Therefore, it lays out treatment guidelines for the care it will pay for and the amount of time it expects to be billed for. Providers who go outside this standardized model to health care delivery will soon be bankrupt. It is therefore understandable that they go along with it or risk being bankrupt and not having their claims paid within a reasonable period of time.

There are a myriad of other penalties and nasty little things the system can and will impose on such providers-- if the provider happens to be competent to address the myriad of problems listed above and tries to do so. The sad fact is that most medical doctors, osteopaths, APRNS, pharmacists, psychologists, and physician assistants are not. That is, most do not have the knowledge of, biochemistry, genetics, epigenetics, lab analysis, nutrition, nutraceuticals, environmental toxins, and how pharmaceuticals actually work in real live patients that is needed, in order for them to be able to sort out the root cause of the problems.

Even those that do have this ability (which is a small percentage of the occupations just listed above, all naturopaths, and most chiropractors) but are working under the third-party payer model of paying for health care services can't invest the time needed to do the sorting. Again, the system makes it nigh impossible for it to be done on a mass scale.

In other words, each of us taking prescription medications is basically on our own-- if we are seeking optimized health, wellness, and longevity. Moreover, those who fail to act may never know what happen because health, post mortem, and other vital statistics are not structured to detect such complex, and often subclinical, cause and effect outcomes. Therefore, biohacking your prescription drugs can act as a first line of defense against nosocomial and iatrogenic diseases.

BIOHACKING AND TAKING PRESCRIPTION DRUGS

The term "Biohack" was first coined in a 1992 Washington Post Article, *Make Way For the Age of The Biohacker and Turbocharged Tomatoes* by Michael Schrage. Since that time, the term has become more and more popularized as evident by the number of google searches.

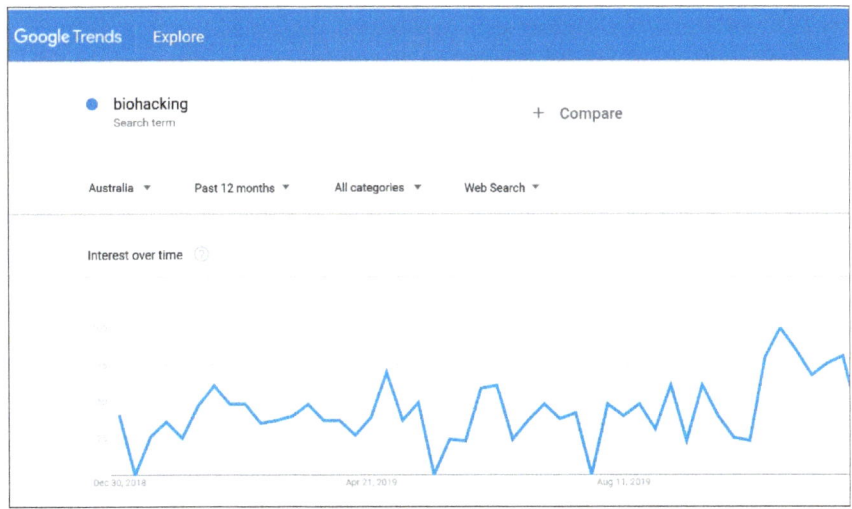

Google Trends *Search trends for the term biohacking: 2004-2018*

The term was controversial when it was introduced in the article and remains somewhat controversial to this day, but what does it mean?

Well, Merriam-webster.com defines biohacking as

Biological experimentation (as by gene editing or the use of drugs or implants) done to improve the qualities or capabilities of living organisms especially by individuals and groups working outside a traditional medical or scientific research environment. The experimentation is often done on one's own body

In an online blog, one author argues that biohacking can be considered a form of self-improvement since it is the practice of changing your body's chemistry and physiology through science and self-experimentation." He further notes, though, that "*the term incorporates a wide range of areas and methods…from something as simple as using nutrition and lifestyle changes to improve how your body functions, to DIY gene therapy, to altering your own body by implanting cybernetic devices…People that modify their bodies in this way are called grinders and, according to the grinder website biohack.me, they "practice functional (sometimes extreme) body modification in an effort to improve the human condition."*

Now, while I don't typically rely on Wikipedia for obtaining information about health, I did in this instance because of the ephemeral nature of the biohacking concept. According to Wikipedia, biohacking may refer to five different areas:

- Do-it-yourself biology, biotechnological social movement in which individuals and small organizations study biology using the same methods as traditional research institutions
- Grinder (biohacking), people that alter their own bodies by implanting do-it-yourself cybernetic devices
- Nutrigenomics, using nutrition to hack/take control of the human biology

- Quantified self, measuring various biomarkers and behaviors to try to optimize health
- Self-experimentation in medicine

We will come back to these ideas shortly when we develop a definition for the phrase *Medication Biohacking* but for now it makes sense to ask, what does it mean to Biohack prescription medications? Before turning our attention to that, however, Lets be sure we are all on the same page when it comes to what I mean when I use a few other common, as well as, medical terms. Having shared understandings about definitions will lay a firmer foundation for understanding the meaning of medication biohacking that I will propose later on in this book.

Drug

We all know that a drug is a substance that has a physiological effect when introduced into the body.

Medicine

We also know that medicines or pharmaceutical preparations are drugs. Drugs are made up of powerful chemical molecules. All medicines are drugs but, of course, all drugs are not medicinal and this difference is a large part of how we have come to think about drugs. Drugs obtained over-the-counter or by a prescription are acquired legally and are assumed to be medicinal. Those obtained through other often illegal means are considered to be street drugs whose use and purchase is illegal. But, the status of a drug can change and fluctuate. Cannabis is an example.

In essence, drugs prescribed by an NP or MD are medicines called prescription drugs. Drugs purchased legally without need for a prescription are called over the counter drugs. Prescription drugs are also called "legend" drugs. Both types are legal and are the focus of this book. That is, we will only address drugs that are in legal category.

Nutraceutical

It is worth noting, however that there is a third type of substance called a nutraceutical or nutrient. Nutraceuticals may or may not be available by prescription and may or may not be available OTC. We will be addressing nutraceuticals later on in this book. For now, however, we want to note two points. First, as a group, nutraceuticals are incorporated into federal law as "dietary supplements" and *as a group* they are also powerful chemical substances—drugs. Second, the pharmacodynamics of prescription drugs often require the need to use nutraceuticals.

Medicinal

Now we agree that a medicine is substance or preparation used in treating health problems or diseases. The term, medicinal, derives from the term medicine and means, "of, relating to, or being a medicine tending or used to improve health, maintain health, treat disease or relieve pain."

Pharmaceutical

A pharmaceutical is simply a medicinal drug. And finally, that said, we now turn our attention to the other key term in our title--medication.

Medication

Once again, we ask, what is it? What is a medication? The not as simple as it might seem answer is that a medication is a medicinal substance, a substance used for medical treatment. Pharmaceuticals are medicinal drugs. By comparison, nutraceuticals are medicinal nutrients or dietary supplements that provide health or medical benefits in addition to their basic nutritional value.

Health

But what is health? It seems that in defining the term medicine, we stumbled upon another important term, the word health. So once again we ask what is it? What is health?

A dictionary definition of health says that health is "*the state of being free from illness or injury.*" The nursing profession's view of health, however, is much broader and <u>starts</u> with the World Health Organization's (WHO) definition of health.

WHO defines health as "*a state of complete physical, mental and social well-being and not merely the absence of disease or infirmity.*" The definition encompasses quality of life and nursing takes things to the next level to include functionality. The nursing profession is married to health, so much so that the American Nursing Association (ANA) defines nursing as t*he promotion and optimization of health and abilities, prevention of illness and injury, facilitation of healing, alleviation of suffering through the diagnosis and treatment of human response to actual or potential health problems, and advocacy in the care of individuals, families, groups, communities and populations.*

Whew! It is obvious that the practice of nursing and the practice of medicine are distinct but overlapping professions. One of the places the two professions overlap is in having independent legal authority to prescribe pharmaceuticals and nutraceuticals for the purpose of promoting patient well-being.

This is true for medical doctors in all U.S. states. But it is only true for advanced practice nurses in about half of the U.S. states. This is because APRNs are not accorded legal authority to prescribe pharmaceuticals in most of the so-called red states where medical associations have persuaded state legislators to keep APRNs status as that of a physician assistant, more or less, rather than the professional advanced practice clinician they are educated and trained to be. Being forced to practice as a midlevel physician assistant poses a powerful barrier to health care access. But, legislators in some states prefer to maintain the status quo, regardless of what it does to their constituents.

Pharmaceuticals or prescription drugs can be very, very powerful substances whose physiological effects can be at times, life giving and health sustaining. On the other hand, they can be deadly or very harmful. Historically, medical doctors prescribed the medications and nurses administered them. Therefore, historically and to this day, medication administration is so important that minimizing any error in that process is of major concern in nursing.

This concern is made apparent in a document called the "Five Rights of Medication Administration." The Five Rights is a list of steps developed by nurse educators for nursing students as a guidance to keep in mind while they are administering medications to their patients. In other words, the Five Rights were developed to help protect patients by serving as a basic defense against medication error. As such, the Rights have been and remain required rote memorization for nursing students.

The "rights" are that medications must be 1) given to the right patient, 2) the right drug—the one prescribed, 3) the right dose, 4) given by the right route, and 5) given at the right time. Over the years, two additional rights have been added. 6) the drug is given for the right reason and 7) the administration of the drug must be followed by the right documentation. Nurses and nursing students now strive to adhere these "Seven Rights of Medication Administration."

They do so out of recognition that the Seven Rights provide a solid fundamental framework for safely administering medications to patients. The Rights are meant to protect patients and understandably revolve around safety and expectations about patient safety. Our discussion about biohacking prescription medications, assumes that the safety expectation is being met. Therefore, we take the discussion to the next level of addressing the issue of medication effectiveness also known as medication efficacy. Although safety and efficacy are related, they are not the same thing. They are, instead, two distinct but overlapping aspects of administering prescription medications.

Medication Biohacking

With all of the above information in mind, we are now ready to define *Medication Biohacking*.

Medication Biohacking is the act of using high quality science, clinical, and evidence-based information to safely optimize the efficacy of medicinal drugs.

We have now concluded defining and discussing key terms that will help you understand the more complex concepts we will be defining and discussing next. Understanding the more complex terms will enable you to implement the 7 biohacks, safely and effectively and give you as much control over your health as humanly possible.

You can use any of the 7 biohacks alone, or with support and guidance from your health care provider, as you prefer. The more of the biohacks that you implement, the more you will benefit. Let's finally see what they are.

PART TWO
THE 7 BIOHACKS

BIOHACK #1
CONDITIONS OF ADMINISTRATION

As discussed earlier, the conditions under which a medication is administered is critical to whether or not it can achieve its therapeutic purpose. Conditions of administration are connected to route of administration but they are not the same things.

So, the first hot hack I'm bringing to your attention is the importance of

knowing the conditions under which the medication should be administered for best effect.

This is not always obvious. That is, depending on the drug and the purpose for prescribing it, routes of administration can be ophthalmological, otic, nasal, oral, nasogastric, transdermal, anal, vaginal, intravenous, intramuscular, subcutaneously, etc. But,

knowing whether or not an oral medication needs to be taken on an empty stomach, with a meal, with or without a meal, or followed by, say 8 ounces of water is also an important condition of administration for medication effectiveness.

Or,

knowing how long a sublingual drug needs to stay in place before other oral substances are consumed is another example of an important condition of administration

You may wonder how can that kind of information be obtained in this super busy, time conscious health care culture? First, the prescriber of the drug should tell the patient or provide a written patient education information sheet that highlights the conditions required for the prescribed medication to be effective. Second, if the drug is picked up from a brick and mortar pharmacy, the pharmacist should apprise the patient of the conditions needed for medication effectiveness along with a written patient medication insert from the drug's manufacturer. Third, the route of administration should be on the medication label. Fourth, the medication can be searched for online at a reputable site, such as WebMD . Fifth, there are a variety of drug reference books available for free use through university and public libraries. Sixth, there are a huge number of drug reference manuals, books, and drug reference apps for use on smart phones. Some are free such as goodRX or drugs.com but others have to be purchased.

BIO-HACK #2

UNDERSTANDING THE PHARMACOKINETICS OF YOUR MEDICATIONS

Okay, so you've just swallowed a medication. What's next? Well, what happens next depends on the form and formulation of the drug you just swallowed. First, as a general rule, drugs in liquid form will process faster than drugs in a solid form. Second, some meds are designed (formulated) for timed release in various parts of the gastrointestinal system or over varying periods of time. Regardless, once the drug has been taken into the body, we enter an arena called pharmacokinetics.

There is a ton of information on the internet about pharmacokinetics. Click Here for a 13-minute introduction to the topic called *"Pharmacology – Pharmacokinetics (made Easy)."* After watching it, check out the AusmedEducation Fast Facts continuing medical education video and graph below.

As you can see, the graph shows major concepts of importance in pharmacokinetics. It comes from AusmedEducation's 3-minute video in which the professor explains each important idea about pharmacokinetics in a very digestible manner. Click Here to view the video.

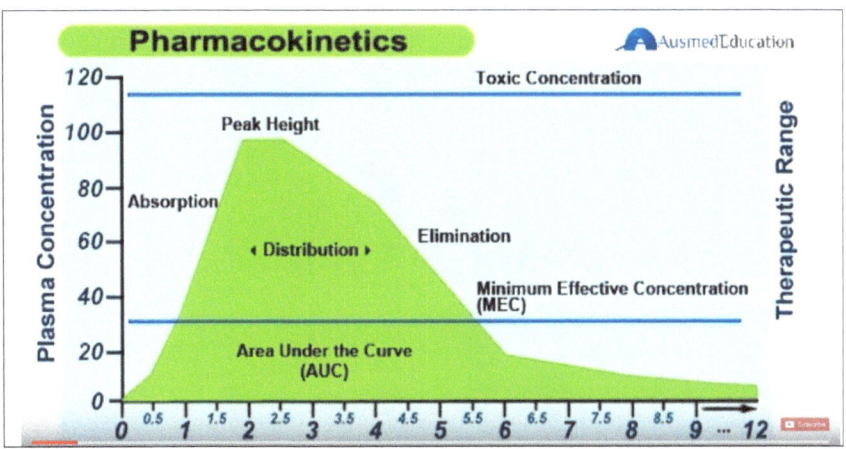

Taken together, the above videos and drawings will help you build a very useful understanding that empowers you to be able to bio-hack your medications very aptly, almost effortlessly with the use of one additional tool.

What is that tool? An up-to-date list of pharmaceuticals that-- But wait, as you will see shortly, there is more.

BIO-HACK #3
UNDERSTANDING PHARMACODYNAMICS

It used to be said that pharmacokinetics was about what the body does to a drug while pharmacodynamics is about what the drug does to the body. According to [Merck Manual](),

Pharmacodynamics (sometimes described as what a drug does to the body) is the study of the biochemical, physiologic, and molecular effects of drugs on the body and involves receptor binding (including receptor sensitivity), postreceptor effects, and chemical interactions.

Whew! That's a mouthful, right? But it is the other half of the piece about what happens once a medication is applied or ingested--taken into the body. [Click Here]() to view a 12-minute lecture on pharmacodynamics from Dr. Jennifer Herndon. [Click Here]() to see what *"Pharmacology - Pharmacodynamics (MADE EASY)"* has to say about pharmacodynamics in a 13-minute video.

[Click Here]() for a quick summary of some of the important concepts in pharmacodynamics. [Click Here]() to view another 3-minute YouTube video that emphasizes additional important concepts.

BIO-HACK #4
KNOWING YOUR PERSONAL PHARMACOGENETICS

Pharmacokinetics and Pharmacodynamics often overlap and nowhere is this more evident than in pharmacogenetics. Pharmacogenetics is concerned with how genetic differences affect our response to medications. Investing in a one-time pharmacogenetics test can be an invaluable biohack.

Why? Well, about 50% of Americans have gene mutations which affect the rate of how they metabolize drugs while 70% have at least one gene variation in the CYP450 system! Based on what we know, the following table presents a concise summary of how the speed of drug metabolism can differ among individuals.

Pharmacokinetic Metabolizer Types and Consequences		
Metabolizer Phenotypes	Active Drug	Pro-Drug
Poor Metabolizer (PM)	• Active drug is likely to accumulate • Lower dose of active drug will be needed to avoid toxicity for buildup	• Inactive prodrug likely to accumulate • Inadequate or no therapeutic response

Intermediate Metabolizer (IM)	• May need reduced dose of active drug to avoid buildups • May cause drug-drug interactions with other medications	
Extensive Metabolizer (EM)	• Standard dose likely adequate	• Likely adequate
Ultra-Rapid Metabolizer (UM)	• Will need higher dose of active drug in order to offset the higher metabolism rate.	• Rapid onset of effect • May require lower dose to prevent excessive buildup of active metabolites

Wise use of pharmacogenetics testing can help avoid up to 95% of drug disposition variability and between from 40-60% of adverse drug reactions!

There are a myriad of pharmacogenetics testing companies and home testing kits are widely available. Beware, however, that many commercial testing companies may not provide the information needed for efficacious drug prescribing. Because of this, pharmacogeneticstics.com an online public interest group advises the public to undertake this type of self-care activity in collaboration with a health care provider. To learn more, check out at Pharmacogeneticstesting.com.

BIO-HACK #5
SELF-MONITORING FOR DRUG SIDE EFFECTS

To monitor yourself for drug side effects, you need to record baseline data, preferably before starting a new medication. This data provides you with a frame of reference in helping to determine the likelihood that the new medication is causing an adverse reaction in you.

BIO-HACK #6

SUPPLEMENT YOUR PHARMACEUTICAL PRESCRIPTION WITH NUTRACEUTICALS

Ok. Now here is something you may find surprising. While prescription drugs are prescribed to help you overcome the symptoms and problems of one or more health conditions, some of prescription drugs can actually harm your health and may even cause deaths. How? The short answer is that they can do so in a variety of ways. One major cause of problems, however, is that some drugs deplete your body of the very nutrients the body needs to maintain its functionality! Loss of those nutrients may mean you never fully heal, heal slowly, or are left in a state of chronic nutrient deficiency and imbalance, or die prematurely. The statin drugs are one example of this phenome.

While not all prescription drugs cause nutrient depletion, the fact that some of them do means you will need to take the time to find out whether the drugs you take affect body nutrients. In other words, in order to protect yourself, you need to discover what essential and nonessential nutrients are affected by the drugs you are taking. You must do it yourself because most health care providers, including pharmacists, don't volunteer this information. Why?

First because most are probably not aware of this adverse effect of the drugs they prescribe. Second, if they are aware, they fail to appreciate the importance of losses, especially compared to all the other more dramatic side effects some drugs can produce. Third, even if a provider is aware of the nutrient depletion side effect, because provider patient encounters are very time constrained, it is easy for a provider to overlook the fact that they failed to tell you about the possibility of nutrient depletions and the short and long-term harm that can result. Fourth, since most health care providers know very little about vitamins and minerals, even if they think about the fact that the drugs, they are prescribing are likely to deplete your body of nutrients, they don't know how to prescribe nutrients for you that can remedy your particular the situation. Therefore, you are on your own.

To help get you started, here is a list of the drug classes that are known to cause nutrient depletion.

LIST OF DRUG CLASSES KNOWN TO CAUSE NUTRIENT DEPLETION

- Acid-suppressing drugs and antacids
- Antibiotics
- Anticoagulants and antiplatelets
- Antidepressants
- Anti-epileptics, aka, anti-convulsant
- Anti-hypertensives
- Anti-psychotics
- Benzodiazepines
- Cholesterol Lowering Drugs, especially statins
- Digoxin
- Diuretics
- Hormone Replacement Therapy Drugs such as estrogens
- Oral contraceptives
- Oral hypoglycemics

BIO-HACK #7

KNOW ALL THE INGREDIENTS IN THE NUTRACEUTICALS YOU TAKE

This, of course means you must read the label on the package. If any part of the ingredients or recommended dosing instructions are covered up by store stickers and the like, you can often get clear uncluttered label from the manufacturer's web site. If this information is not on the web site, it is probably a good idea to choose another brand. But, don't take the nutraceutical until you know what is in it!

Avoid taking nutraceuticals that have used inorganic herbal ingredients. Inorganically grown herbal ingredients have often been found to contain lead, pesticides, like Round-up, and other toxins. Moreover, plants grown inorganically are often grown in soil that is largely depleted of the natural organic (including microbes) and mineral matter found in healthy soil. Therefore, plants grown in such soils are unlikely to have the natural nutrient power needed to achieve medicinal effects.

EPILOGUE

There you have it. You now have the basic knowledge framework to begin to start working on biohacking your prescription drugs safely, consistently, and easily. It will feel awkward at first but hang in there and remember that the longest journey begins with the first step.

If you would like additional support, feel free to sign up for membership in Scsson's free membership plan. Scsson is the health and wellness arm of Mind Body Works Telehealth and, as shown in Part III, Scsson offers subscription self care support services.

The Basic Plan is designed for those who would like to:

- Receive weekly mailings of our flagship Newsletter, "This Week's Body Measures" (TWBM).

- Learn more about using nutraceuticals to optimize health, and

- Purchase competitively priced pharmaceutical grade nutraceuticals with free shipping on orders costing $50.00 or more.

Scsson supports you in your self care efforts *whatever* your current level of wellness. Again, Scsson's Basic Membership Plan is free. [Click here](#), or go to [www.scsson.com/scsson-subscriptions](#) to sign up.

Whether you decide to go it alone, work with your regular health care provider, or subscribe to an online self care service support plan, like Scsson, please *do start* working on implementing these 7-solid biohacks. They can greatly improve the efficacy of the drugs you take while improving your overall health and wellness helping you have a healthier longevity.

Happy Hacking!
NP Dr. Olivia Young

PART THREE
PUBLISHER AND AUTHOR NOTES

ABOUT SCSSON

Scsson stands for Self Care Support Services Online. Scsson's goal is to be the premier telehealth self care support service on the internet.

Scsson is part of the private practice model of prescribing advanced practice registered nurse (APRN) nurse practitioner (NP) clinician, researcher, publisher, and author, NP Dr. Olivia Young.

According to her. the idea for Scsson stems from the melding of her prior education and experience with her work as a travel provider.

As a travel APRN-NP who has practiced in two east coast two west coast, three central and one southern U.S. states. Regardless of where I practiced, I repeatedly witnessed ill-health, disability, and premature demise strongly tied to preventable causes. Sadly, health care systems seem ill-prepared to remediate the situation. Therefore, I've decided to try to help patients by providing actionable self health care information to the public through Self Care Support Services Online (Scsson) Publishing. 7 Prescription Drug Biohacks: Hot Bio-hacks That Can Help You Increase Your Medication's Effectiveness" is the second book Scsson has published. However, it is my first self-help health care book written to specifically support actionable self care activities.

As suggested above, before starting this publishing and writing venture, I worked full-time as an APRN NP, researcher, and educator in my private telehealth practice and as a travel health provider for a variety of temporary staffing agencies. My formal education is in nursing, nursing education, applied research, and political science. My post graduate education and clinical work has focused on computing, addictions, using whole food nutrients and nutraceuticals as medicine and integrating their usage with pharmaceuticals when appropriate, longevity, healthier living, and anti-aging theory and practice.

Scsson offers a five-level self care support service by subscription. Scsson also conducts health and other research and publishing relevant to self care and optimizing health and longevity.

ABOUT THE AUTHOR

NP Dr. Olivia L. Young is an advanced practice registered nurse (APRN), board certified psychiatric mental health nurse practitioner (PMHNP-BC) whose practice specializes in integrative telehealth care, addictions, and wellness oriented psychiatric mental health.

She has been an APRN since 1981 at which time, she specialized as a family nurse practitioner (FNP). She has been a registered nurse for over 40 years and also has extensive research and university teaching experience in nursing education and applied research methods.

In addition, she has helped to launch a number of innovative patient-centered health care ventures such as This Week's Body Measues Newsletter, Mind Body Works Telehealth (www.mindbodyworks.us), Psych Meds Online (psychsmedonline.com) and Self Care Support Services Online (www.scsson).

Her email contact is: npdryoung@scsson.com.

SCSSON'S SELF CARE SUPPORT PLAN

Mind Body Works Holistic Integrative Care
Subscription Membership Plans

Our Free Basic Subscriber Plan
The Basic Plan is designed for those who would like to receive weekly mailings of our Flagship Newsletter, This Week's Body Measures" (TWBM). TWBM is chock full of mind-body health information that can greatly support readers' own self-health care efforts.

Shipping Costs; Free (Email Delivery Only)	Annual Dues Free	Monthly Dues Free

Our Bronze Subscriber Plan
The Bronze Plan is designed for those who
1. Would like to receive weekly mailings of our Flagship Newsletter, This Week's Body Measure" (TWBMs) and
2. Would like the ability to make unlimited periodic purchases of pharmaceutical grade nutrients (PGN) such as vitamins, minerals, amino acids, nutritional substrates, etc., at current retail market prices.

Shipping Costs; Free for orders over $50	Annual Dues $59.00	Monthly Dues $4.99

Our Silver Subscriber Plan
The Silver Plan is designed for those who
1. Would like to receive summarized evidence-based self-care health information
2. Is already spending $50 a month or more on Over-The-Counter (OTC) supplemental nutrients for active self-care or treatment.
3. Would like to upgrade the quality of the products they use by only purchasing valid and reliable research evidence-based food and pharmaceutical grade nutrients, and
4. Would like to be able to consistently obtain such nutrients at discounts up to 10% off the current retail pricing.

Shipping Costs; Free for orders over $50	Annual Dues $120.00	Monthly Dues $9.99

Our Gold Subscriber Plan
The Gold Plan is designed for those who
1. Would like to receive summarized evidence-based self-care health information
2. Is already spending $50 a month or more on Over-The-Counter (OTC) supplemental nutrients for active self-care or treatment.
3. Would like to upgrade the quality of the products they use by only purchasing valid and reliable research evidence-based food and pharmaceutical grade nutrients, and
4. Would like to be able to consistently obtain such nutrients at discounts up to 15% off their current retail pricing.
5. Would also like to be able to have access Self-Care Support Services (SCS) consisting of 1 annual online consultation about their health, one free bridge prescription annually, and lab* ordering as indicated

Shipping Costs; Free for orders over $50	Annual Dues $239	Monthly Dues $19.99

Our Platinum Subscriber Plan
The Platinum Plan is designed for those who
1. Would like to receive summarized evidence-based self-care health information
2. Is already spending $50 a month or more on Over-The-Counter (OTC) supplemental nutrients for active self-care or treatment.
3. Would like to upgrade the quality of the products they use by only purchasing valid and reliable research evidence-based food and pharmaceutical grade nutrients, and
4. Would also like to be able to consistently obtain such nutrients at discounts up to 20% off their current retail pricing, and,
5. Would also like to have access to Total Integrative Care
   Total Integrative Care Services consist of
   - an initial complete intake evaluation, diagnosis, treatment, lab ordering and follow-up as indicated. and/or referrals with follow-ups as indicated.
   - 2 free online consultations about their or their loved one's health annually,
   - 35% discounts off the costs of consultations numbering more than 2 in a 12-month period
   - two free bridge prescriptions in a 12-month period and
   - personalized health education consisting of recommended articles readings

Shipping Costs; Free for orders over $50	Annual Dues $599	Monthly Dues $49.99

MAY I ASK YOU A FAVOR?

If you found this book interesting, or have found any benefit from reading it, will you please post a review of it on Amazon?

Few things excite me more than new reviews, especially reviews that suggest new topics readers would like me to write about. I read all reviews and they inform my future writing.

So, if you are willing to take 5-10 minutes to write what you sincerely think about this book, please visit 7 Prescription Drug Biohacks' Amazon page and post your opinions.

Best regards and thank you!
NP Dr. Young

FREE BIO-HACKING TOOLS ON THE INTERNET

Here is a Link to The Entire FDA Drug Safety and Availability Web Site. It is huge and a bit overwhelming.

However, the following two links can be very useful in your quest to successfully bio-hack your medications. Here's what I suggest you do:

1. Download FDA's Free 3-Page Glossary of Terms Relative to Drug Safety FDA Guide to Drug Safety

2. Check Out and bookmark FDA's Free Searchable Medication Guide Database. It takes time to get use to using it but doing three searches, it will seem like a drop in the bucket.

SEND QUESTIONS, SEND FEEDBACK

Please feel free to send any questions or feedback directly to me.

SEND TO: npdryoung@scsson.com

or

prescriptiondrugbiohacks@scsson.com

I WILL TRY MY BEST TO RESPOND IN A TIMELY MANNER.

NP DR. OLIVIA L. YOUNG

www.ingramcontent.com/pod-product-compliance
Lightning Source LLC
Chambersburg PA
CBHW040332220526
45473CB00009B/2657